Get Your Shape Back In 37 Days

You Will Find It Surprisingly Simple, Just Learn To Eat The Right Food And Stay Fit For Good

Table of Contents

Introduction

Obesity is itself the biggest problem because there are lots of diseases associated with the obesity. An obese person may suffer from mood swings, depression, fatigue, irregular menstruation, constipation, migraine, etc. It is not easy to reduce weight because people hate diets and workout. People don't like diets because a traditional diet means to cut out all of your favorite food items to reduce calories. You may feel deprived and felt miserable. The situation is not new because everyone finds it difficult to start a strict diet by cutting their favorite food.

It is the biggest misery that the weight may come back as you stop dieting. Everyone tries to do dieting at least once in his/her life because more than 60% Americans are overweight and 30% are categorized as obese. The figures are increasing at a rapid rate in the rest of the world. Now the question arises that why people are gaining so much weight. Is it because of overeating or the reason is different. It is the fact that nowadays, people are eating less fat as compared to the people in the past.

Just visit a grocery store, and you may notice numerous foods with "Low-fat, Zero-Fat, Free from Fat and Low calorie" tags. Restaurants offer diet soda, low-fat meals, and low-calorie desserts. The saturated fats are replaced with fake fats and the sugar is replaced by the artificial sweetener. You can conveniently get low-calorie and fat-free food items, but still you are getting fatter more than before. What is the reason behind this?

It's simple to answer is that a low-fat diet is not effective for you because these are full of artificial contents instead of natural ingredients. These ingredients are not healthy and promote weight gain instead of weight loss.

The book is designed for your help so that you can dramatically get your shape in 37 days. The diet program is specifically designed for your help and after reading this book, you will find that there is no need to cut your favorite food items, desserts, and snacks because a healthy and balanced diet plan is designed for you.

Chapter 1 – Understand Your Body and Metabolism

Fat is essential for your body because it can make your food tasty, and you will surely feel satisfied after every meal. It is also important for the growth and nourishment of your body. Your body may store fat to get energy for the long-term and short-term needs. The fat is essential for the vital organs and to protect your nerve cells. The fats you eat prove helpful in the digestive process and increase your metabolism rate in the form of triglycerides. There is a natural way through which the human body digests food and following are some steps through which the digestion and metabolism works:

Mouth and Stomach

The digestion of fat may start from the mouth because there are some glands under the tongue that secrete enzymes like lingual lipase and Gastric lipase. These are important for the stomach to work with the molecules of fats. The stomach works on the molecules of the fat because the walls of the stomach may act like a blender to churn and mix the food items. This can blend the fat by breaking in the smaller ones. The stomach may take more time to digest fats as compared to protein and carbohydrates. The meals with higher fat contents will keep you fuller for the longer periods of time.

Small Intestine

The fat digestion starts as your food travels to the small intestine from the stomach. The upper part of the smart intestine is known as the duodenum, and this part can act mechanically on the fat to emulsify it and the bile acids are released from the gallbladder. The bile acids are produced by the liver and stored in the gallbladder. The pancreatic lipase is a secretion of the pancreas to tear the triglycerides into monoglycerides, diglycerides, and fatty acids.

Absorption and Movement of the Fat

The fat components are then absorbed in the lining and walls of the small intestine. The short-chain fatty acids may have 14 carbon atoms that can straightly access the portal vein to bind the protein albumin and travel to the liver to use as energy. It can be converted into a longer chain. There are 14 or more carbons that can transform into the triglycerides that may convert into chylomicrons. These chylomicrons are sent slowly to through the lymph stream and then released into the blood stream.

Metabolism (Energy and Storage)

The chylomicrons pass through the blood stream to distribute the triglycerides into tissues as per its requirements. These can be fats, muscle tissues, and adipose. The 20 percent of the triglycerides are delivered to the liver in the broken parts so that the liver can produce energy after absorbing them. Fatty acids are important for your cells to produce energy except brain cells, eyes, and red blood cells. The fatty acids are converted into a substance through a beta oxidation process. This substance is important to create a carbohydrate metabolism.

Know your body (Body Mass Index, What does your BMI mean and what is the 'ideal' weight)

BMI means body mass index and it is calculated on the basis of the weight and height of a person. It is a reliable indicator to know about the fitness of the body. BMIE does not mean the direct measurement of the body fat, but it is a correlation of the body fat measures. It is a cheap method to screen your category of weight to treat it because excessive weight can lead you to different health problems.

What does your BMI mean?

Body mass index is a defined measure used by the physician and experts to know the status of your weight either you are underweight, overweight or obese. The BMI number will give you a clear indication of your health and well-being:

BMI	Result
Below 20	Underweight
20 - 25	Healthy
25 - 30	Overweight
30 and Above	Obese

Calculations of the BMI

The BMI of the adults and children are calculated with the use of the following formula:

- Formula: weight (kg) / [height (m)]2 where the measuring units can be Kilograms and meters (or centimeters).

- Formula: weight (lb) / [height (in)]2 x 703 for the pounds and inches measuring units.

The Devil (What Calories are and the causes of weight gain)

Calories are the unit of energy that you consume on a regular basis. Calories mean consumption of energy through food items and drinks. The energy is required to perform different physical activities. For instance, an apple has 80 calories and a tablespoon of sugar may contain more than 100 calories. If you want to walk 1 mile, you may require energy equals to 100 calories. There are two types of calories:

- Small Calorie: Its symbol is cal and the 1 cal is the amount of energy required to increase the one gram of water by one degree Celsius.

- Large Calorie: Its symbol is Cal, Kcal and it is equal to the amount of energy required to increase the one KG of water to a degree Celsius. It means 1 large calorie (1kcal) = 1,000 small calories

Some people consider that only food and drink has calories, but the reality is quite different. Everything that can give you energy has calories. The calories are quite important for the human body because you can't survive without energy.

Human body cells require energy; similarly the heart, brain and lungs may stop working in the absence of energy. You can get the necessary calories from food and drink to supply energy to your body.

By consuming a limited amount of calories on a regular basis, you will be able to live a healthy and happy life. The food items contain different amount of calories and it helps you to determine the energy your body will get by consuming each food. There are three main components of the food, like protein, fats, and carbohydrates.

- 1 gram protein can give you 4 calories

- 1 gram fat comprises of 9 calories

- 1 gram carbohydrate may contain 4 calories

It means 24 grams fat can give you 216 calories, 30 grams protein may give you 120 calories and the 2 grams carbohydrates may provide 8 calories to your body.

Chapter 2 – Understanding the Basics of Weight Loss and Healthy Food and Traditional Meal Plans

Balanced Diet?

A balanced diet should be an excellent combination of vitamins, minerals, carbohydrates, proteins and other important content. The diet should base on the scratchy food items like rice, bread, fruits, vegetables, dairy foods, milk, salt, sugar and other important items in a balanced proportion. Taking a healthy and balanced diet means enjoying a variety of food items in the right proportion and consume the right amount of food and drinks according to the requirements of your body.

Food Groups in the Balanced Diet

Eat well to maintain your health and avoid obesity and other relevant problems. A balanced diet should contain:

- Lots of fruits and vegetables

- Different types of scratchy foods like rice, pasta, potatoes and bread

- Meat, beans, eggs, and other food items should be in your regular diet to get sufficient proteins

- Enjoy milk and dairy food items

- Small amount of food and drinks with fat and sugar

It will be good to include different types of food items in your regular meal and have enough amounts of vegetables, meat, fruits, fat and sugar to keep you fit and active.

Ideal Food items for the Balanced Diet

The balanced diet should have vitamins, minerals and other important nutrients with low fats and sugar. Following should be included in your balanced diet:

Fruits

Fruits can be taken as healthy and quick snacks because these are full of important nutrition. You can get seasonal fruits of your areas to get all important nutrients.

Vegetables

The essential vitamins and minerals can be obtained from the dark and leafy vegetables because these can help you to consume nutrition at every meal. You can get the advantage of delicious, spinach, beans, broccoli, cabbage collard greens and kale.

Grains

The grains are important for your body because these contain a maximum amount of nutrition. The grains are available in the form of rice, bread and pasta.

Proteins

Proteins are really important for your body because you can develop the good brain, muscles and decrease your body fat. The proteins can be obtained through chicken, fish and other animal meat. If you want to reduce the cholesterol in the meat, it will be good to remove the skin to reduce the fat.

Tofu, tempeh, and soy-based products are rich sources of the protein. These are healthy alternatives of meat and you can get all important proteins for your body through natural food items.

Know your food (what are good fats/carbs, bad fat/carbs)

Before eating food, it is important for you to know your food. There are different food choices available for you that may include good fats and carbohydrates and bad fats and carbohydrates. It is important to understand the different between good and bad fats and carbohydrates. Your food should be a right combination of the vitamins, minerals, good fats, carbohydrates, proteins, etc. The people often can't recognize the difference between the good and bad carbohydrates. Some carbohydrates are really bad for your health and you should avoid them. It is significant to fill your regular diet with the real food. You can make some healthy choices like brown rice instead of white rice and orange juice instead of vitamin water.

Good Carbs and Bad Carbs

- The good carbs are fresh fruits, vegetables, and whole grains. The food should be low in the calorie density because the good carbohydrates may increase your satisfaction level.

- These should be high in healthy nutrients

- Refined sugar may contain 20 percent of your regular calories and the unrefined carbohydrates can affect your metabolism. Consumption of refined sugar can increase the chances of obesity and type 2 diabetes. The white sugar can be directly included into your bloodstream to increase the risk of diabetes.

- Try to consume food items high in natural fiber because it can maintain your blood sugar and insulin level. This can also be the reason in the decrease of the LDL bad cholesterol. The fiber rich food may contain fewer calories and enable you to lose weight at a faster rate. There are lots of benefits of consuming high fiber food because it may help you to get rid of constipation and cancers. The 12 to 15 grams of the fiber on a regular basis will help you a lot.

- Try to take food with low sodium and saturated fat.

- Your food should contain zero fat or less amount of fat to avoid weight gain.

Bad Carbohydrates

- High-calorie food should be avoided like a corn dog and energy bars has lots of bad carbohydrates.

- Refined sugar, corn syrup, and white sugar are added in the canned juices. Avoid them as much as possible and try to replace sugar with honey.

- White flour has refined grains and it has lots of bad carbohydrates

- The food is low in many nutrients

- There is no need to consume food that is low in fiber

- The food with high sodium should be avoided

- The high cholesterol and Trans fats should be avoided

Try to include good carbohydrates in your regular diet because these will help you to reduce excessive weight and maintain a good health.

Good Fat and Bad Fat

Fats and carbohydrates should be an important part of your diet because of their nutritional value. There are lots of choices, but some fats are really good and others are bad to avoid. You should recognize the good fat and bad fat to plan a healthy and balance diet for you:

Good Fats

Following are some good fats that are really beneficial to maintain a healthy cholesterol level and healthy heart:

There are some Good fats that you can consume:	
Available Monounsaturated fat	**Some Polyunsaturated fat**
Oil made of canola	Healthy oilof soybean
Extra virgin oil based on olives	Good oil based on corn
Oil obtained from the sunflower	Safflower oil
Oil made of healthy nuts	Walnuts
Sesame oil	Sunflower, pumpkin and sesame seeds
You should include Avocados in your diet.	The Flaxseed can be included in the milkshakes and smoothies.
Whole olives will be good for you.	Seafood, such as tuna, salmon, sardines, mackerel, trout and herring
The nuts are good (all types of nuts), pecans, cashews, etc.	Soymilk
Peanut butter	Tofu

Saturated Fats and Trans Fats

The saturated fats and trans fats are taken as bad fats and these should be avoided in your regular food. Following are some saturated and trans fats that are not good for your health:

These Saturated fats should be avoided	These Trans fat are not good for you
Red meat with high fat content	Commercial items like cake, muffins, pizza, pastries, doughnuts, etc.
Chicken with its skin (It can be consumed without skin)	Crackers in the packet, popcorns, chips and other food items of the similar food group
Dairy products, such as cream and full-fat milk	Margarine with lots of bad fat
High-fat Butter	Shortening of vegetables
High-fat Cheese	Fried fish, chicken, potatoes and nuggets
Ice cream	Fatty and sugary candy bars
High-fat coconut oil and palm oil	
Pig fat, such as Lard	

Different types of food items are available for you, but it is your duty to carefully choose food items. There are different kinds of food items that will help you to feel satisfied, increase your energy level and maintain good health. The above-given food choices will help you to understand which kind of food is good for you. If you want to decrease excessive weight and increase positive energy, it is compulsory to avoid bad fat and carbohydrates because these can ruin your overall health. Switch to good fats and carbohydrates to increase your metabolism, promote excessive weight loss and reduce negative effects of unhealthy food items on your health.

Chapter 3 – Necessary Foods for Weight Loss and Essential Habits for weight loss

Lots of food choices are available for you, but these choices may contain good food and bad food. The good food items are just like your best friend because these can help you to maintain good health and get rid of excessive weight. There are some important food items that should be included in your regular diet to promote weight loss:

Necessary Foods for Weight Loss

Physical activity and a well-balanced diet are always required to maintain your health and promote quick weight loss. In order to do exercise, your body needs fuel and the food is an instant source of fuels. It means, if you are trying to follow a strict weight loss routine, then it will be difficult for you to have sufficient energy for the exercise. The natural sugary food items and complex carbohydrates can increase the metabolism of your body. If you want to increase your weight loss speed, then it is important to include following food items in your regular diet:

Fiber

At least 20 grams of fiber should be included in your regular diet and you can consume whole grains, vegetables, and fruits to get 20 grams fiber. The fiber can satisfy you for the longer periods of time and you can enjoy its benefits while you are trying to lose weight. The fiber can increase your energy and decrease the risk to gain weight and bad cholesterol in your body. The fiber may be equal to ½ pounds less body weight. The high fiber intake can reduce your total calorie intake and increase your weight loss speed.

Calcium and Vitamin D

Calcium and vitamin D works together to increase the strength of your body. If you want to make your weight loss successful, you should include dairy foods in your regular diet. Vitamin D can promote weight loss because it can act with the leptin hormone. You can take supplements of vitamin D and calcium to avoid deficiencies in your body. If you are trying to lose weight, then it is important to include enough supplements of 1000 IU of the vitamin D. It is recommended that the men and women of the 19 to 50 years should take 1,000 milligrams calcium, and the men and women of 51 or more age should take 1,200 milligrams.

The regular recommendation of the Vitamin D is almost 200 IU for the 19 to 50 years men and women. The men and women between 51 and 70 years should take 400 IU. The men and women of the 71+ should take 600 IU.

Good Fats

If you are trying to lose weight, it is important to consume good fats because the Omega-3 fatty acids are good for you to consume. You should include avocados, fish, nuts and vegetable oils in your food. You can take almost three to four servings in a day. The good fats will increase your weight loss speed and reduce bad cholesterol. It is important to take 1,300 milligrams of the omega fatty acids in a day. It will reduce your hunger and provide lots of health benefits.

Protein

Almost three servings of the lean protein should be included in your diet. The lean protein means fish, chicken, white meat, pork loin and turkey. It is essential for your body and keeps you full for the longer period of time. Try to take high protein in your breakfast to have a good start for your day. It will increase your metabolism and weight loss speed.

Water

It is proved by some researchers that the water is important for your body to increase your energy, calorie burning speed and metabolism. There are numerous benefits linked with water because the water will keep your body free from toxins and maintain the health of your kidney. Water is an excellent substitute of the sugar drinks, soda, flavored milk and energy drinks. You should include almost 10 to 12 glass water in your daily routine.

If you want to increase your weight loss speed, it will be good to drink at least 3 to 4 glasses of water in the morning before taking breakfast. This may help you to enjoy numerous health benefits. You can add a lemon in water to enhance its taste, but don't include sugar and salt.

Green Tea

Almost 3 cups of green tea are important to include in your regular routine because the caffeine in the green tea will reduce your belly fat. The green tea is an excellent drink to lose weight. It will be good to drink almost 2 to 3 cups of green tea without sugar and salt. Add a lemon in a cup of green tea to increase the fat melting speed.

Essential Habits to Lose Weight

If you want to promote weight loss at a good speed, following are some essential habits that will surely help you:

Dieting is Not Good

People usually start quick diets to quickly reduce weight, but they should understand that it is not a good habit to reduce weight with a strict diet. It can augment weakness of your body. It will be good to change your lifestyle and add healthy food items in your diet. Replace bad and fatty foods with healthy and natural food choices.

Set your Weight Loss Goals

Your weight loss can be easy and consistent by setting some practical weight loss goals for you. The goals should be practical enough to follow because these can increase your motivation to work on a goal to get successful results. For instance, having a goal to lose 30 pounds in 30 days can be a dream, but reducing 5 to 10 pounds in 30 days is a practical goal.

Reward Yourself

After accomplishing each goal, you should reward yourself because it can encourage you to do more to get more. Keep it in mind that food is not a good reward for you. It will be ideal to try a movie, entertainment show or a spa treatment as a reward.

Understand Portion Size

Portion size plays an important role to determine the success of your weight loss. If you want to increase your weight loss speed, you should control your portion. Choose a small plate to eat food and fill your plate with healthy choices. You can maintain a food diary to control your portion size.

Chapter 4 – Set your goal (how much weight loss is normal/healthy)

There are lots of diets available to lose weight, but it is important to consider a safest and healthiest way for you. Before setting your weight loss goals, you should determine how much weight loss is normal and healthy for you. The healthy way to lose weight at a faster rate should be based on the principle to burn more calories than you eat. Your calorie consumption and its burning rate may determine the weight loss speed. If you are trying to lose weight fast, you can increase your activity level to make your work more efficient.

Healthy Weight Loss

The experienced health professionals have suggested that you can reduce almost 1 to 2 pounds in a week and it is a safe range. If you want to increase your weight loss speed, you should be careful about the combination of calories and exercise. Reduce your calorie intake and increase your regular exercise to lose weight in a healthy way. It will help you to determine your weight loss goal.

Reduce your Calorie Intake

If you want to reduce one to two pounds in a week, you should cut the 500 calories from your regular consumption. It may base on your diet to cut the high amount of calories. You can increase your portion size by including low-calorie food in your diet and decrease your portion size if you want to consume high-calorie food. If you want to increase the speed to achieve your goal at a faster speed, you should drop almost 1050 to 1200 calories in a day. You can follow a

1,200 calorie diet to increase your weight loss speed. It will help you to come closer to your ideal weight. A diet and exercise plan is essential for you and following are some easy ways to reduce your calories:

- Reduce your portion size, use a smaller plate to feel fuller

- Low-fat versions of food are available

- There is no need to take creamy and fatty sauces. You can prefer healthy vegetables and vinegar instead of sauces

- Additional fat in food items should be replaced with healthy fats

- Snacks should be replaced with fresh fruits and popcorns

- Think about your eating choices and write about bad things to increase your awareness.

Set Your Weight Loss Goals

If you want to increase your weight loss speed, try to set your own goals, but these should be practical enough. Unpredictable goals will not help because you may not be able to reduce 15 pounds in a week and it may lead you to disappointment. Try to establish practical goals so that you can enjoy good results. It is important to get rid of the harmful exercises, pills, and plans because these will not help. Increase the consumption of healthy meals and include a good physical routine in your lifestyle to achieve your weight loss goals.

How mental health plays a role?

Motivation is really important for the person trying to lose weight because it will be a signal that you are doing something good and to get its long-term effects you should keep following it. Your good mental health will help you to make your weight loss easy. If you are interested in getting rid of extra pounds, you should be very strong on your weight loss goals. There are some mental strategies that will help you to avoid overweight problems:

Think Thin

If you are trying to lose weight, starts thinking that you are a thin person and you have to reduce weight to look sexy and pretty. Visualize your image of six months after that try to feel that you are looking good by shedding some extra pounds. Change your lifestyle and try to break all bad habits to increase your success rate in the weight loss.

Design Realistic Goals and Expectations

Realistic expectations to lose weight can increase your motivation because the realistic goals are easy to achieve. There is no need to consider that you will lose 20 pounds in a month because the average weight loss ratio is 1 to 2 pounds in a month.

Set Small Goals

If you want to increase your weight loss speed, try to use the power of your mind and make a list of smaller goals to achieve them. You can increase your motivation in this way. It will make your life easy, like:

- You can think to eat more fruits and vegetables in a day

- Involve in a kind of physical activity for almost 30 minutes in a day

- Enjoy alcohol only on weekend

- Eat low fat popcorns to replace fried food

- Use a salad instead of fries

- Use stairs instead of lift

Get Support of your Family Members

If you want to increase your weight loss speed, it is important to tell your friends and family members about it to get their support. It will help you to strictly follow your goals and enjoy each and every benefit of the physical activity and healthy eating.

You can use your will power to increase your determination to reduce weight. Stick to your plans and carefully follow every health plan. You can eat nuts and good food items to increase the power of your brain.

Chapter 5 – Portions and Seven Day Exercise Plan

There is a difference between the portion size and serving size because portion means to pile on your plate and the serving means using a standard. You should choose small spoon and serving plates to control your serving size because it helps you to reduce the calorie intake. You can choose a small plate, cup and spoon to limit your portion. A big half plate will not satisfy your craving, but a small full plate can help you to control your hunger. There is no need to skip meals because you can eat as much as you can, but for this purpose, your plate should be filled with the healthy fruits and vegetables.

Try to make your plate colorful by adding fruits, vegetables, meat and grains in it. You can use a small bowl and spoon to increase your satisfaction. An ideal portion could be comprised of healthy food items. Following are some quantities of food items that make one complete serving:

- 1 cup raw vegetables or chopped fruits are equal to one serving

- 1/4th cup of cooked veggies is equal to one serving

- A whole fruit of 4 ounces equals to one serving

- 6 ounces fruit juice equaling to one serving

- 1/4th cup dry fruits mean one serving

- 1-ounce cheese is one serving

- ½ can tuna or chicken salad makes one serving

- 2/3 serving cup of yogurt is one serving

- 2/3 cup milk means one serving

- 3 ounces potato makes one serving

- 1-ounce bread slice means one serving

- 1 waffle or pancake means you have one serving

- 1/3 cup rice and quinoa mean one serving

- 1/3 cup cooked pasta means 1 serving

- 2/3 cup cereal makes one serving

- 1-ounce chips make one serving

- 1 teaspoon butter makes one serving

- 1 tablespoon nuts make one serving

- 4 ounces poultry make one serving

Seven-day Exercise Plan with sets of exercises

Exercise is really important to reduce an excessive amount of weight because in order to get rid of excessive weight, you should burn excessive calories from your body. It is important to do enough exercise to burn more calories and the amount of exercise may also depend on your goal to lose weight. There is a sample seven day plan with sets of exercises. You can try them as it is, or make some changes in the plan according to your availability of time and physical strength.

Monday Workout Plan	In the Morning
	<ul><li>10 jumping jacks</li><li>10 high knees</li><li>10 heel kicks</li><li>10 calf raises</li><li>10 tuck jumps</li><li>10 walking lunges</li></ul>**In the Evening**<ul><li>10 squats</li><li>10 push ups</li><li>10 leg raises</li><li>10 crunches</li></ul>
Tuesday Workout Plan	<ul><li>Push-up (Upper Body): 10</li><li>Abdominal crunch (Core): 20</li><li>Total body Step-up onto chair: 10</li><li>Triceps dip on chair (Upper Body): 10</li><li>Plank (Core): 30 seconds</li><li>Lunge (Lower Body): 10</li><li>Push-up and rotation (Upper Body): 10</li><li>Squat (Lower Body): 10</li></ul>
Wednesday Workout Plan	<ul><li>20 jumping jacks</li><li>20 high knees</li><li>20 squats</li><li>10 push ups</li><li>10 leg raises</li><li>10 walking lunges</li><li>10 crunches</li></ul>

Thursday Workout Plan	• 20 calf raises • 30 second plank • 20 mountain climbers • 20 back extensions • 20 push ups • 20 bench / chair triceps dips
Friday Workout Plan	• 20 jumping jacks • 20 high knees • 20 heel kicks • 20 squats • 10 back extensions for your back fat • 10 leg raises • 10 bicycle crunches • 10 push ups
Saturday Workout Plan	• 10 Burpees (with a push up) • 10 Crunches
Sunday Workout Plan	• 50 to 100 high knees / running in place • 50 to 100 pushups • 50 to 100 sit-ups • 50 to 100 squats

Note: You can follow this routine on a weekly basis, such as start this routine from Monday again after finishing one week.

Conclusion

Weight loss is really difficult with traditional methods, but now lots of crash diets are available for your help. There are lots of drawbacks and problems attached to these diets. You may face serious health threats. If you want to reduce weight without any weaknesses and long term effects, you should combine everything in your diet.

The good news is you can create a diet plan with maximum food to avoid starvation. Your diet plan should contain a balanced combination of all important things to avoid starvation and deficiency of anything. There are some exercise plans and diets that may help you to get rid of weight.

FREE Bonus Reminder

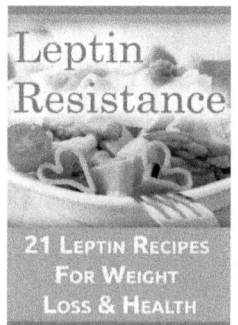

If you have not grabbed it yet, please go ahead and download your special bonus report *"Leptin Resistance. 21 Leptin Recipes For Weight Loss & Healthy Living"*.

Simply Click the Button Below

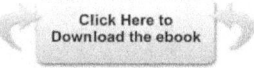

OR **Go to This Page**

http://easyweightlossway.com/free/

BONUS #2: More Free Books

Do you want to receive more Free Books?

We have a mailing list where we send out our new Books when they go free on Kindle. Click on the link below to sign up for Free Book Promotions.

=> Sign Up for Free Book Promotions <=

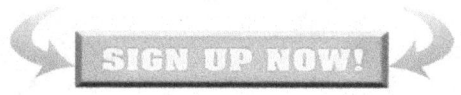

OR Go to this URL

http://bit.ly/1WBb1Ek